Healing Ourselves
Naturally

A Practical Guide towards a
Vibrant, Fulfilled Life

Charles Stone
Monika Schneider Stone

HEALING OURSELVES

Contents

FOREWORD

CHAPTER 1
WAKING UP

CHAPTER 2
OUR DAILY BREAD

CHAPTER 3
A SPIRITUAL PRACTICE

CHAPTER 4
METAMORPH-OSIS

CHAPTER 5
ENCOURAGEMENT

CHAPTER 6
RE-TREAT YOURSELF

CHAPTER 7
WATER...WATER...

CHAPTER 8
COMMUNE WITH NATURE

CHAPTER 9
HEALTH ASSURANCE

CHAPTER 10

MANIFESTING A RICH LIFE

CHAPTER 11
PASS IT ON

CHAPTER 12
GRATITUDE

Why We Wrote This Book

A Major Shift in Consciousness is Happening Now on Earth...

Our Planet and all it's inhabitants are beginning to experience a powerful shift in consciousness. What many know to be the Aquarian Age or the age of breaking out of the collective unconscious... the organized, controlled way of life... what some call the 'Matrix'. Approximately every 25,000 years, the Earth goes through a different cycle which corresponds to whichever constellation it is moving towards. The cycle we are now moving out of is the Piscean or the age of the ego, hierarchy, self-centeredness, greed, and so on. For around 2,000 years, humans and other beings have been under the influence of authoritative and manipulative, male dominated societies. Everyone was expected to behave and perform a certain way and to 'conform' to the ways of society.

Ancient Secret Wisdom in the arts of Spiritual Awareness and Natural Healing were largely hidden from the general populace and used by those in power to try and control the masses. But now in this age of Aquarius, the wisdom of the Ancients is being revealed through growing numbers of people waking up to this new energy. At the same time the old, archaic systems are collapsing and a whole new consciousness is emerging... Spiritual and Physical Sovereignty. We finally begin to understand that we do not need anyone or anything outside of ourselves to save us. We realize that we are already 'Saved'... already whole within ourselves. We are becoming free from the bonds of control and 'Societal Desensitization'. In other words, the collective unconsciousness.

Establishing and maintaining a higher level of awareness can be accomplished by following the guidelines in this book.

In this age of information and technology, we have instant access to practically all that is happening at any time, anywhere in the world. Most of what is reported is unsettling news. We can easily get emotional about some event or other which we feel is unjust or unfair. Not just here in our own land but in other parts of the world. We must be vigilant to not take any of what we see or hear from the mainstream media seriously. We need to be careful to not allow the fear or anger of the collective unconscious affect us in any way. As difficult as it may be to accept, let us trust that everything is happening just as it is supposed to. Understand that all the chaos and madness which is occurring now is symptomatic of the shift into the Aquarian age.

However nothing is ever just 'Good' nor is it only ever just 'Bad'. Remember that although it oftentimes does not appear so, both energies are arising simultaneously. And... Everything at it's extreme turns into it's opposite.

So have Faith... Maintain Hope... the time is coming where all wars will stop and Peace will prevail on the earth. Kindness, Love and Compassion will overtake greed, selfishness, and hatred. But it begins with us...

Heal Yourself. Each and every one of us has the inherent ability to change our own lives... to heal ourselves and maintain a vibrant conscious awareness. The illusion that others somehow control us or have taken away our power to live a free life is... Simply not possible. Your power can never be taken away for it is who you are at your very essence. Once we realize this... that we are in control and always have been, then we stop blaming our outside circumstances and the world. Immediately we give up the role as the victim and regain our freedom... Our Physical and Spiritual Sovereignty. We discover that we alone are responsible for our Health, Happiness, and... our Grace.

Light up your life. Create a brilliance within and without through your dedication to transforming yourself and everyone around you. Become a beacon of light... an inspiration for positive change and healthy, vibrant living. Transform the world... one being at a time just by being yourself... An example of pure, exhilarating life force. One person can change many. A few can change all of humanity. As you walk this path, you will naturally attract to you more and more people who are also waking up... who are shifting their consciousness and embracing the emerging heart energy. Work together. Know that you were destined for this... Teaching, healing, serving, and loving all beings of our world.

If you are reading or hearing these words, then the brilliant light of awareness is already beginning to shine within you.

'A wise person knows intuitively that health is the greatest of human blessings'. Hippocrates

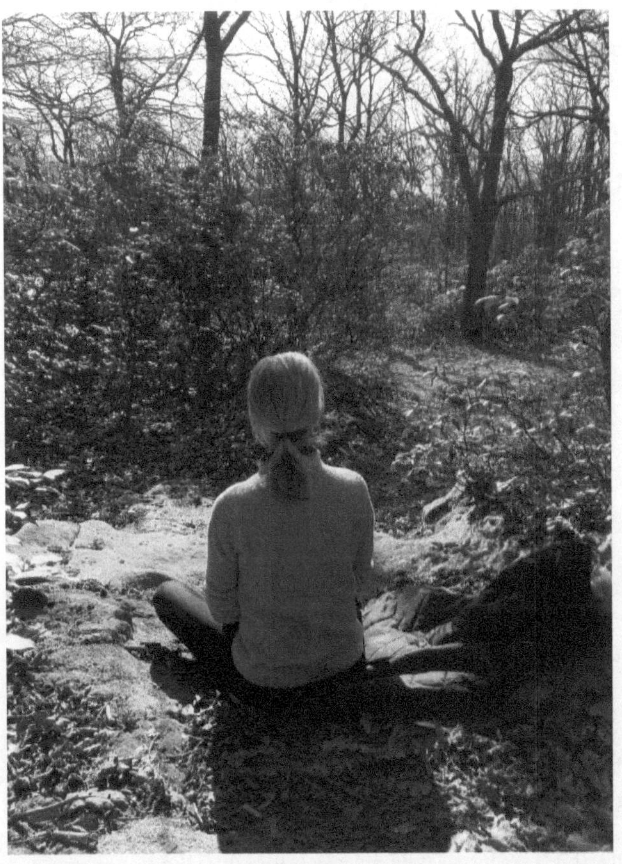

Foreword

$\quad$ This little book is written with the intention to be a guide and inspiration for anyone wishing to make healthful, life enriching changes. The essence of these writings are based on the authors' personal life experiences. This book is not intended to be a 'How To' Reference or Manual. There are already so many great books available on Alternative Health, Diet, Whole Foods Cooking, Spiritual Practices, Appropriate Exercise, and other self help subjects. Instead, what we offer you are tidbits of wisdom and inspiration to point you in the right direction towards self-healing. Here is an opportunity to awaken what you already possess - that inner spark of 'intuitive knowing' which lies dormant, waiting ever so patiently, to be recognized and nurtured. For many of us, all we lack is some direction and a bit of inspiration.
Here we share with you a recipe for a way of life filled with vibrancy, abundance, contentment, and of course, great health. Gathered from our own personal life experiences, we offer you this practical, common sense wisdom in the hopes of pointing you in the right direction to start you on your path to self-healing. Once you are on the path, the rest is up to you. Trust in your good judgement and your inner intuitive abilities.
We wish for you that you choose to follow this 'Awakening' towards, not only self nourishment, but the

inevitable healing influence you will have on your family, friends, and community.

This can be, perhaps, your most remarkable life's journey yet... Perhaps challenging - nevertheless joyous.

A journey which will surely change your life... for the better... forever.

If your intuition has now led you to this little book, then you are already on the path towards self-healing and... if after reading it, you choose to embark on this remarkably transformative journey then... 'May the Force' be with you'.

In Peace and Love, Charles Stone & Monika Schneider Stone

CHAPTER 1   WAKING UP

That magical moment. The mysterious, ethereal 'gap-in-time' when we emerge from deep sleep into the world of consciousness... how sweet and delightful it can be when welcomed by thoughts and feelings of pure gratefulness and a smile on your face.

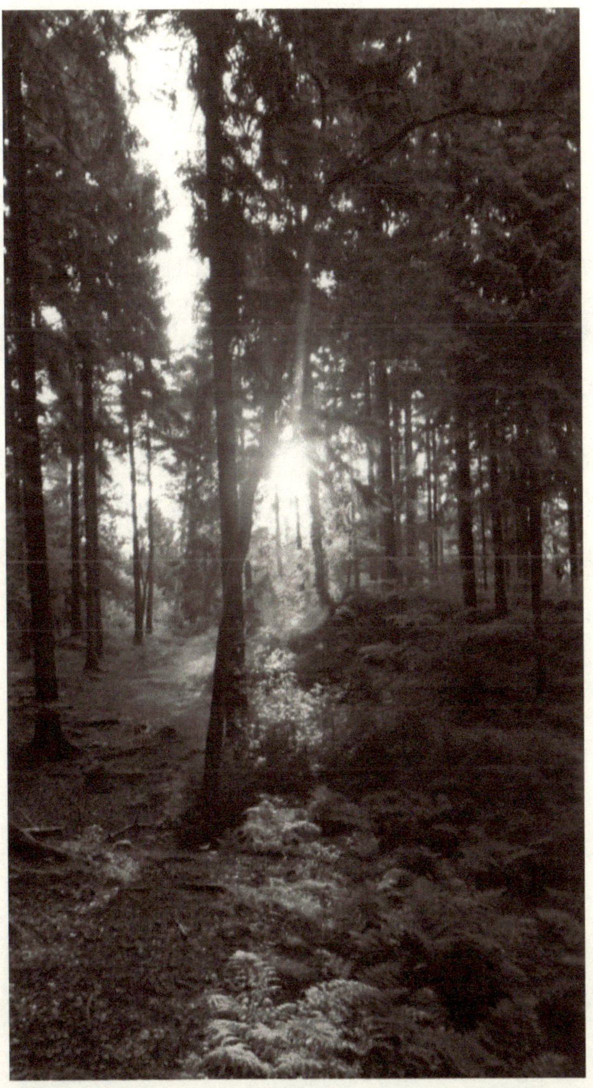

Our very first thoughts in the morning are essentially the seeds we plant for how our day will 'unfold' and…

whether we experience life as a joyous experience or a burdensome, arduous trek.

Waking up out of sleep with feelings and thoughts of deep, heartfelt gratitude for another day to experience life as a human being on this Earth is a glorious blessing.

There are those who would say, 'This is impossible in this stress-filled world'. But I can promise you from my own experience and diligent practice, it is indeed possible to consciously change negative, energy draining thoughts into positive, nourishing ones. And over time, you will jump out of your bed like a young child on Christmas morning.

Each and every one of us possess this ability to develop into grateful, happy beings. Patience and courage are needed however, the rewards are beyond belief and are boundless.

Breath Awareness

This means simply realizing that you are, in fact, breathing. The breath is something precious that we often just take for granted. In reality it is truly all we have, but many of us are barely conscious of how our breath controls virtually every moment of our lives. Conscious breathing can bring us into a place of presence and with it better focus and expanded awareness. Deep breathing sharpens our intuition therefore creating mindful decision making and a closer, more intimate relationship with ourselves, those around us, and our environment.

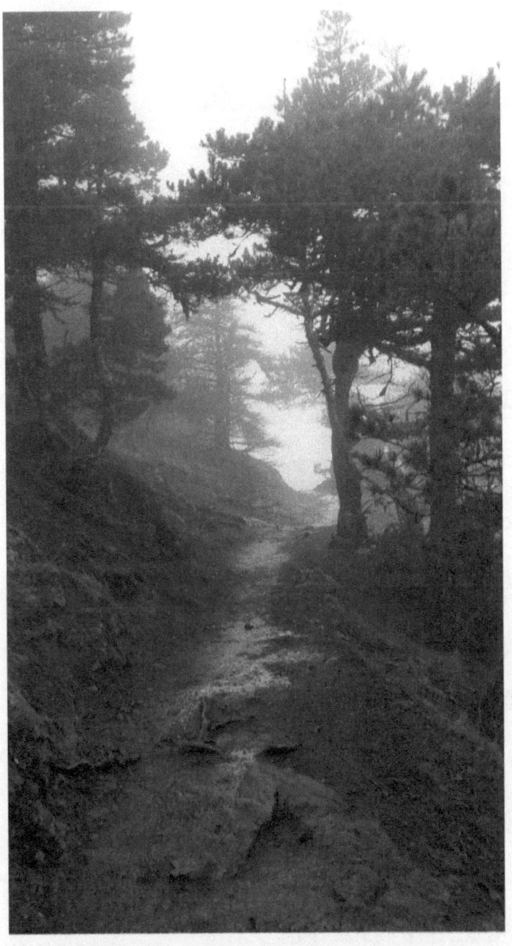

Every morning, as you rise and make your bed up, practice simple deep breathing with a long, slow inhale and a long, slow, full exhale. Begin slowly and softly (so you do not pass out on the floor). Remember that you just spent hours of very shallow breathing and you might easily become lightheaded. Continue this conscious breathing exercise as long as you wish for the next ten or fifteen minutes as you go about your morning. You will be amazed at the benefits.

Cold Shower

Nothing stimulates that **I'm Awake!!** feeling like an icy cold shower.

The next most important part of your morning wake up is a refreshing, cold shower.

I am not yet as brave as my wife, Monika so I simply rub down my body with a coarse brush and then jump under cold running water for as long as I can stand it… usually two to three minutes. Monika scrubs her entire body with a coarse bath brush followed by rubbing an organic, neutral (non-perfumed) body oil over her skin. Standing under icy cold water in the shower she rubs again with the coarse brush.

Some may think of this morning ritual and shudder with frosty thoughts. . Others say they wish they had the time for this. Personally (and from my own direct experience) I do not feel this is a valid excuse for not trying this amazing, life invigorating ritual... and here is why.

This morning routine greatly improves circulation and combined with brushing, nourishes and invigorates the skin as well as stimulating the lymphatic system. The little know, but highly important Vagus nerve is given attention that under normal circumstances is neglected. The Vagus nerve has powerful influence over our entire health. It is connected to most of our vital organs and when stimulated, boosts the immune system as well as digestion.

 In addition, our skin has become softer, smoother and more elastic. Any skin imperfections have all but disappeared. Our body's natural temperature regulator actually returns to a normal state… and a glowing warmth spreads over you and stays with you throughout the day. This is a welcome benefit for those of us who chill easily in the cold winter months. Yes, just because it is minus ten outside and snow is lying on the earth does not mean you go back to hot showers.

The feeling of aliveness does not stop with the vibrant, eyes wide open sensation on the physical body. We have, both of us, increased our mental clarity and alertness. 'Relaxed Focus', I like to call it, has become an integral part of our personalities.

If you are still not convinced, consider the fact that the oldest living humans on Earth begin their day with a cold shower. On the island of Okinawa, for example, where many do not even have the luxury of hot, running water, they are among the longest living beings on the planet.

Besides all of the above mentioned benefits, you will save money on your water, gas and/or electric bill... because, let's face it, who wants to linger under an icy cold shower.

A wonderful and nourishing 'after shower drink' is a cup of hot herbal tea with fresh squeezed lemon or, if you have a juicer… fresh, organic juice. Our favourite is carrot-apple-ginger juice. This juice combination gives you the vitality to get you through your morning exercises until breakfast.

CHAPTER 2   OUR DAILY BREAD

'Medicine is not Healthcare. Eating natural foods is Healthcare. Medicine is 'SickCare'. Let us finally understand this distinction.' Anonymous

A Unique Diet for Everyone

As many people as there on planet Earth is how many different diets that may exist. All humans have a unique combination of constitution and condition. Add to this, environment, age, daily exercise, profession, including many more factors and we begin to understand the complexity of attempting to 'Universalize' a dietary regime. Simply put, there is no one specific diet for everyone. Developing our intuition and instinctive abilities enables each of us to customize the perfect diet for our personal lifestyle. Fortunately, from years of research and experimentation, there are many sample diets and reliable recommendations now available.

In America, the sixties and seventies gave rise to numerous alternative dietary lifestyles… Vegetarian, Raw Foods, Macrobiotics, Vegan and various other fad diets.

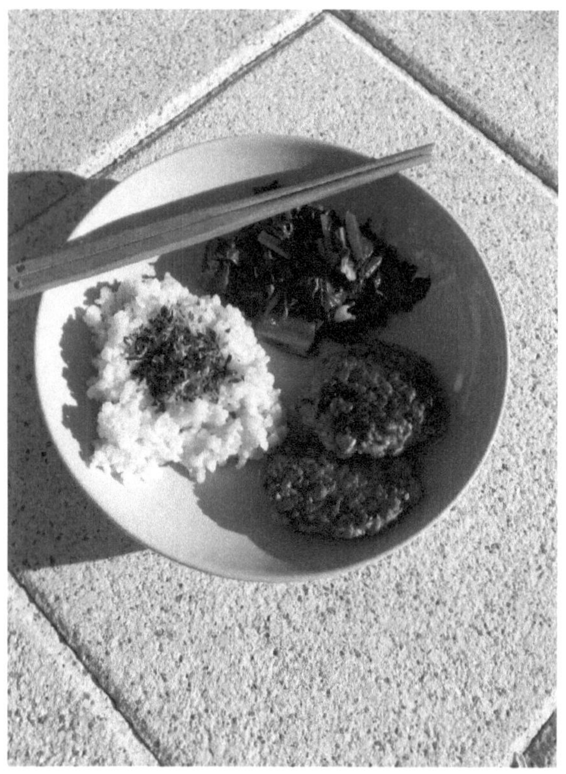

Among those which have survived to the present time are Vegetarian(ism), Vegan(ism), and Macrobiotics

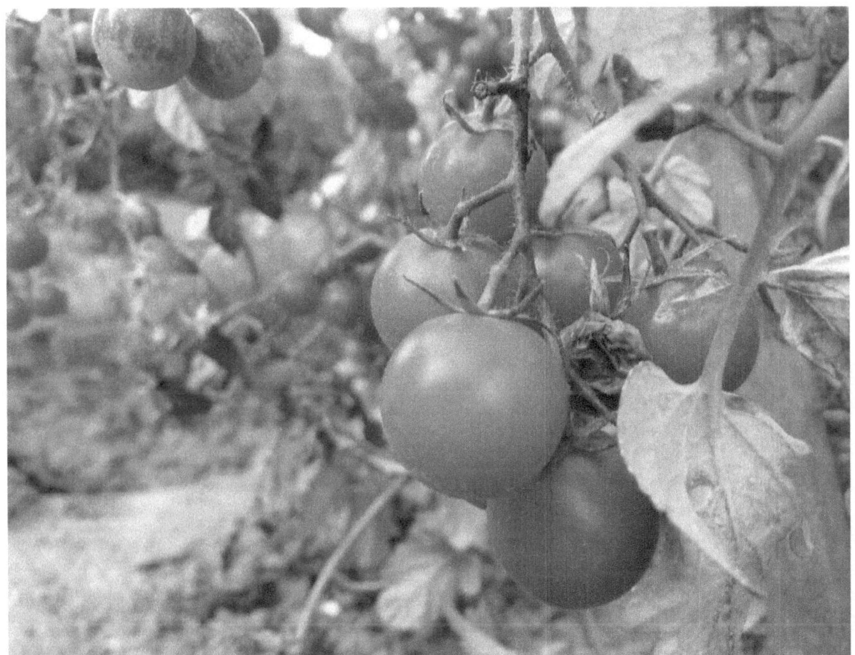

Vegetarian(ism)

A Vegetarian is referred to as a person who does not eat meat, and sometimes other animal products for moral, religious, or health reasons.

Vegetarians have been on the planet since before recorded history. Some Anthropologists claim humans were 'Gatherer/Hunters before they were Hunter/Gatherers. More recent well known Vegetarians were George Bernard Shaw, Albert Einstein, Benjamin Franklin, and Leonardo da Vinci.

Francis Moore Lappe's book, Diet for a Small Planet, published in the early seventies led to the increased popularity of Vegetarian(ism) in America. Its popularity has increased greatly over the years and continues to draw more and more converts from a meat based diet. Many professional athletes have adopted a plant based diet for increased endurance and stamina. The are numerous benefits for becoming a Vegetarian and this requires some thorough research to insure an informed and healthy transition.

Vegan(ism)

One who embraces a Vegan way of life seeks to exclude, as far as is possible and practicable, all forms of exploitation of, and cruelty to, animals for food, clothing or any other purpose.
One thing all vegans have in common is a plant-based diet avoiding all animal foods such as meat (including fish, and shellfish), dairy, and eggs as well as products like leather and anything tested on animals.

Film stars such as Woody Harrelson, Zooey Deschanel, Brad Pitt, and Joaquin Phoenix all claim to be Vegans (to name a few). The US Representative, Dennis Kucinich, and even former US President, Bill Clinton are said to be Vegan. Professional athletes Tom Brady, Kyrie Irving, and Venus Williams adhere to a Vegan diet and attribute their superior athletic performances to this way of eating.

John Robbins, of the well known, family owned Baskin-Robbins Ice cream franchise is famous for his bestselling book, Diet for A New America, which is a startling examination of the food we consume in the United States, and the astonishing moral, economic, and emotional price we pay for it. This vastly popular and educational book helped launch the Vegan movement in America and inspire a generation to reform their meat consuming diets to a plant based diet.

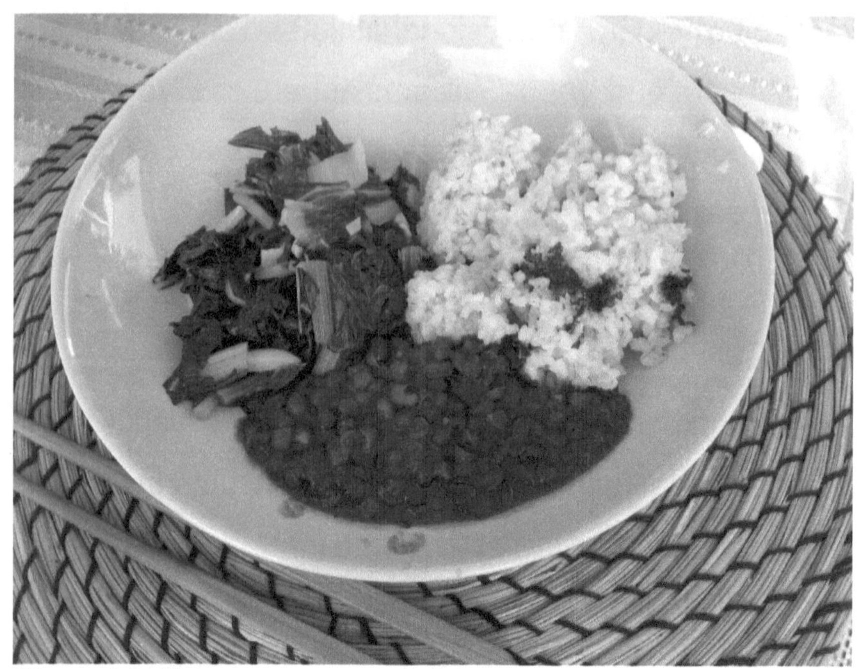

Macrobiotics

Macrobiotics was introduced initially in the US by Michio Kushi having been instructed by his teacher, Georges Oshawa to bring this way of life to America. Based on the definition of the word Macrobiotics; Great Life, the basic premise is that anyone who is truly happy and healthy is considered to be Macrobiotic regardless of their diet. Macrobiotic philosophy centers on vibrant health and longevity through lifestyle principles. The main focus is a grain and vegetable based diet including unrefined regional foods, little or no animal products, and recognizing food selection, preparation, and eating as a healing art. Macrobiotics has evolved over the years and presently resembles a Vegan diet while continuing to include Sea vegetables, Miso, Tamari, and other Japanese specialty foods.

The ancient Chinese philosophy of Yin and Yang is incorporated into these teachings. In essence, all phenomena can be interpreted by Yin and Yang. There is really nothing esoteric about Yin and Yang as it simply explains day changing into night, youth into age, or one season into the next. The Yin/Yang principles, when applied towards an awareness of personal factors necessary for complete health can result in harmonious and creative adaptability. A very brief introduction of Yin and Yang principles; Yang is active while Yin is passive. Yang represents Heaven, Masculine energy, Heat, and Expansion. Yin represents Earth, Feminine energy, Cold, and Contraction, to name a few. Numerous books are available for further study on this ancient theory of life.

'Everything in Creation is covered by Heaven and supported by Earth.'
The Yellow Emperor's Classic of Internal Medicine

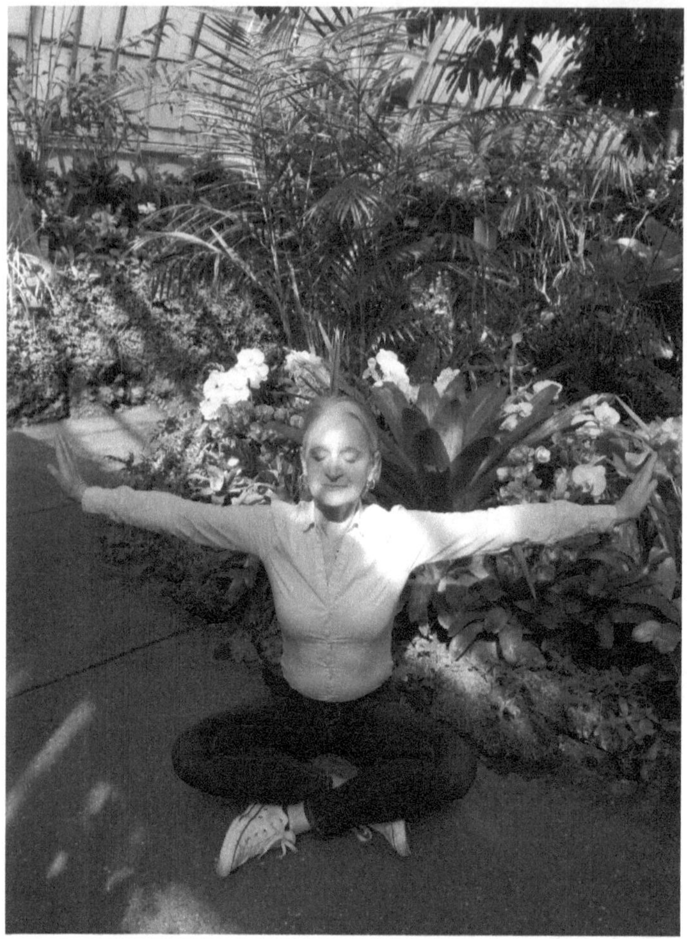

Embracing a new and particular way of life can be fun especially if it is free of any strict philosophical 'Dogma'. Changing our diet and therefore our way of life can be an exciting, educational, and enlightening experience. When we adopt a new way of nourishing and healing ourselves with enthusiasm and enjoyment, the benefits will be astonishing, not only for ourselves but for those around us as well.

It is recommended, to make the transition easier, to develop a basic understanding of the principles of Yin and Yang. You will therefore be able to choose a diet which is customized for your particular constitution and condition.

Virtually every being on the planet could benefit and flourish with a plant based diet. Variations according to individual constitutions and conditions need to be considered as well as age, climate, environment, activity, and profession.

Begin with the basics and what has proven effective for thousands of years. You

can always modify as you go.

Having whole, unprocessed grains as the staple food is optimal supplemented with local, seasonal, and organically grown vegetables and fruits. Beans such as Kidney beans, Adzuki, Black beans, Lentils, and Soybean bean products such as traditionally processed Tofu and Tempeh are recommended for daily use.

Sea vegetables provide essential minerals, vitamins, and amino acids and are an especially excellent source of iodine, calcium, and iron.

Many wonderful Vegetarian, Vegan, Macrobiotic, and Whole foods cookbooks are available to learn about the preparation and cooking methods used in a plant based diet. As long as you have the desire and continue your daily practice, you will naturally and intuitively attract to you what is right for you at this time.

Trust in those who have gone before you and who have for thousands of years not only thrived but flourished eating a plant based diet and were some of the most remarkable cultures ever on planet earth. Taking into account that as modern peoples we have evolved into a markedly different 'Species', we still maintain that a plant based diet can provide the same remarkable results for us. Trust in this. Believe in your own intuitive abilities and... Listen to your body. Your body knows what you need.

'Let food be thy medicine and medicine be thy food.'
Hippocrates

CHAPTER 3   A SPIRITUAL PRACTICE

With Self Discipline almost anything is possible.'
Theodore Roosevelt

Healing ourselves encompasses not only healthy, nutritious food for our physical bodies but also for our spiritual bodies. No matter what your lifestyle is or how demanding, there is still the possibility for making the time for a daily LESP… 'Life Enriching Spiritual Practice'.

Yoga, Meditation or other similar disciplines are remarkably effective in increasing flexibility, strengthening the immune system, reducing anxiety, and boosting energy levels… to mention only a few benefits. However, to be optimally effective, we must be disciplined and practice daily. The longer we continue with a daily discipline, the more powerful our physical and spiritual bodies become and… Even a few minutes of yoga or other discipline in the morning and before sleep are beneficial. It is essential to first decide what it is you want to change in particular about yourself. In this little book, We have chosen to emphasise natural healing of body and mind, therefore our focus will be on exercises which contribute directly towards this discipline.

Yoga as a daily spiritual practice

Witnessing my wife, Monika's enduring optimistic attitude, great sense of humor, and enhanced inner and outer beauty, I finally became inspired enough to participate in her morning Kundalini yoga routine. Through her insistence, I kept at it long enough to feel, at first subtle, but then extraordinary changes . And after having committed to this morning discipline of yoga and meditation for several months, there is no doubt it will now be an integral part of my life.

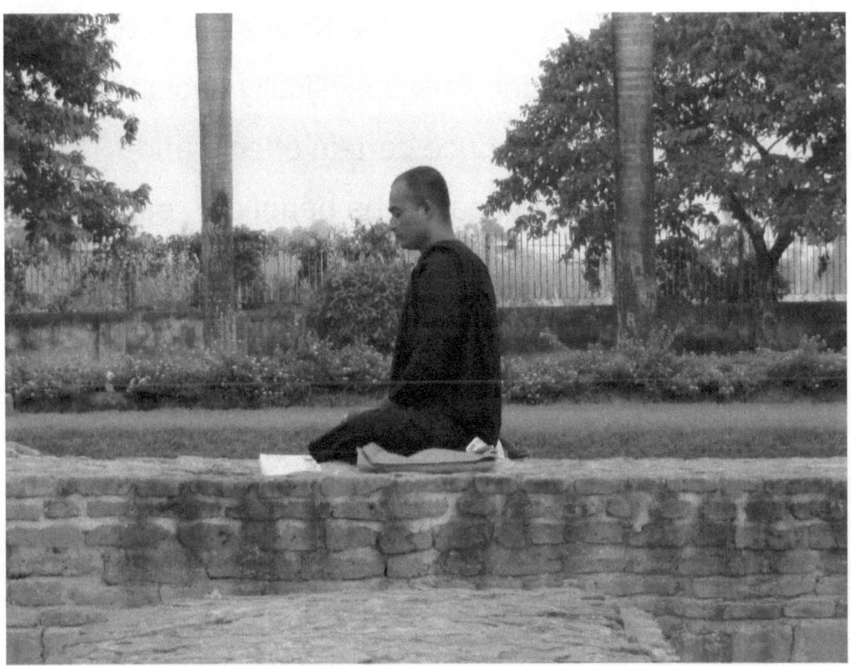

The amazing health benefits of a daily practice of Kundalini Yoga are too numerous to mention here, but I can say, because I have seen through experience, truly remarkably benefits in my physical, mental, and spiritual health, that this style of yoga could improve anyone's health and well being.

That being said, we all have differing needs and what may work for one of us may not necessarily work for another. So many styles of yoga are now available to us that you are sure to find one which resonates with your personal needs. However, if you feel you want to try Kundalini yoga, it is essential that you find an experienced teacher because the Kriyas (sets of exercises) being taught were specifically designed by Rishis and Yogis to produce certain effects and benefits. Any style of yoga will be beneficial, especially when you make it a daily morning practice.

Discover what best works for you and then stick with it. Join a class. Watch videos. Don't be afraid to take advantage of the modern technology which is so readily available to us now. The Internet and the myriad of Yoga, Meditation, and other helpful videos are of tremendous value.

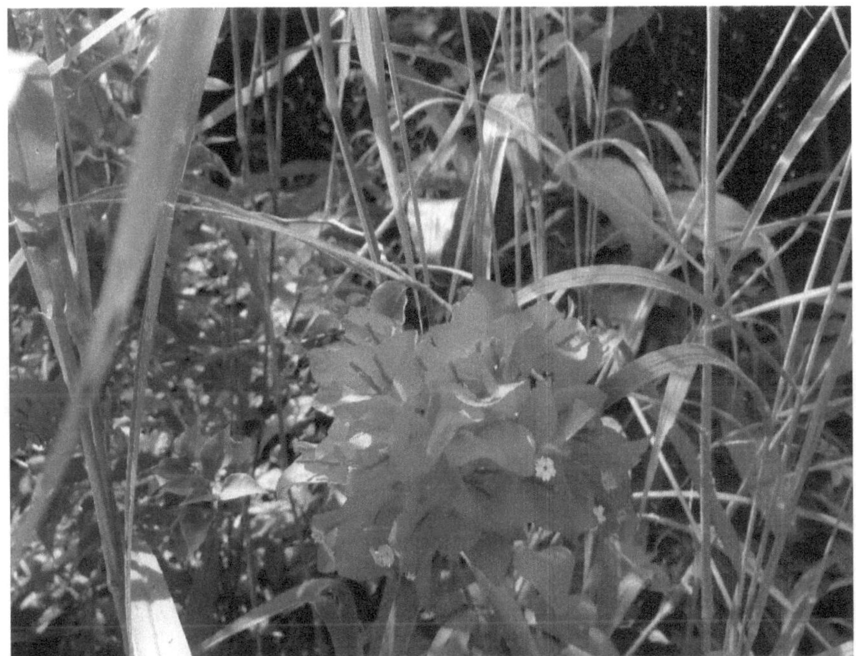

Only a few short months ago, my mornings began with sipping a hot cup of espresso, while I perused the Web anxiously checking the previous evenings sports scores. The intention to institute a morning discipline of yoga or jogging or… something more enriching than sitting in front of the laptop drinking espresso was always somewhere in the back of my mind. I kept promising myself that one of these days I would change my habits. Well… one of these days has finally arrived. Four months into my morning practice of one hour or more of Kundalini yoga and meditation has change my world for the better… Still I am only just a beginner but I feel more vibrant and alive than I can remember. One by one old, non-nourishing habits are being replaced with life-enriching new ones. Additionally, I have developed more patience and understanding. My heart is opening and I am less critical or judgmental of others and... My gratefulness for life is increasing daily and I vow to never take this for granted.

Once you yourself witness the remarkable changes in your life after only a few weeks (out of a whole lifetime) of a daily practice of yoga, meditation or other discipline, you will experience miraculous results and wonder what took you so long to begin.

'Discipline is choosing between what you want now and what you most want.' Abraham Lincoln

CHAPTER 4   METAMORPH-OSIS

'It takes courage to let go of the familiar and embrace
the new.'
Author Unknown

'Metamorphosis is a change of the form or nature of a
being into a completely different one, by natural or
supernatural means.'

from the Greek root translated as...
Meta - 'after or beyond'
Morph - 'shape, form, or structure'
Osis - 'process or action'

One of the most fascinating examples of complete and absolute transformation is the life stages of a butterfly. Particularly the chrysalis stage. Chrysalis translated from the ancient Greek word, khrusallis, (khrusos) means 'Gold'… 'because of the golden colour of the pupae of some species of insects'. I believe this to be a mis-translation. A more accurate translation (at least in my way of thinking) would be because of the pure, fresh, new life which emerges from this complete transformation… literally, from one being into another. This quality of complete transformation is not exclusive to the world of creatures. We as humans possess this capacity of 'Metamorphosis' as well. In the spiritual realm… but also in the physical body. Most often what is required for this to happen is a sudden extreme or catastrophic life changing event. However, this does not have to be. There are alternatives to experiencing the inevitable pain and suffering which normally accompany a tragic, life changing event.

Change is Good

Changing on the outside is for most of us not as difficult as changing on the inside. An exercise routine, a new diet, a physical makeover are all easy compared to deep inner transformation. Dramatic inner change can be as simple as a shift in perception, that is, a new way of interpreting the world around you.

Self discipline and dedication are two important ingredients in the recipe for positive life transformations. What a virtue to have the ability to do this on our own. Acceptance, Enthusiasm, and Enjoyment are other essential components for this self-transformation to occur.

Once the 'Force' of fresh, vibrant energy is coursing through your body and oxygenating your entire being, you will be excited to get started but you will need a plan of action for your 'Life Changing Strategy'. Before you go through your whole home and begin filling boxes with refrigerator and kitchen cupboards, throwing out all your packaged and de-naturalized food items, stop and consider the potential consequences of altering your diet from one day to the next. A sudden and dramatic modification of ones daily dietary habits can result in severe reactions, both physical and emotional. Unless you consider yourself somewhat of a warrior and strong enough to weather these potentially uncomfortable side effects, then it is best to be gentle with yourself and proceed slowly. Here is a brief sample of what one may expect.

Healing Reactions: Changing from the inside out
Here is a wonderful opportunity to resolve and heal anything from our past which we still carry needlessly in our beings. These must be completely cleared out for a total healing to take place. Traditional Japanese medicine says if there is no Meigan (healing reaction) then there is no cure. Proceed wisely and be gentle and kind to yourself. A lifetime of excess cannot be cured in a few weeks.

Physical discharges such as skin eruptions, unpleasant body odour, halitosis (bad breath) may occur as well as nasal and vaginal discharges. Headaches, fatigue, and tension or pain in the neck and upper back are common. Digestive problems, including gas and cramps may also arise. Don't be too concerned for this is only temporary. Many experience weight loss as a direct result of switching to a plant based diet. Depending on your body's level of toxicity, symptoms could disappear quickly or linger on for several weeks. If you are suffering too much or are in pain, incorporate some of your food cravings to slow down the healing process. In the long run, you will be amazed at how great you feel. Of course, as you evolve and change, your dietary needs will change. This is where your developing intuition comes into importance. You will be in tune, body and mind working together, and solutions will present themselves and your progress will be effortless. Relieving uncomfortable reactions on the body are simple and easily applied.

A hot sea salt bath relaxes and soothes tight muscles and tense joints.

Emotional Reactions

Emotionally, most of us feel we are fairly balanced, but wait until you start skipping that morning Espresso, the weekend barbecue or that late night chocolate bar. Mental anguish, cravings, anger, irritability, impatience, and perhaps depression may occur. Wild dreams are also one of the possible mental side effects from changing to a plant based diet. But don't take any of these seriously. You've been carrying these unnecessary emotions around long enough and have been expertly stuffing them. Allow them to surface and just watch. These are perfectly normal side effects of switching from a toxic, unhealthy diet to a fresh, whole foods diet.

Psychological Reactions

Our mother's favorite recipes and cooking methods are still with us as adults whether we realize it or not. This is one of the most difficult psychological attachments to let go of. As a result of facing this reality and having the desire and willingness to leave these comfort foods behind, some forms of depression,

sadness, and melancholy may arise in us. Our cells are actively encoded with these emotional 'attachments' and will take some discipline and courage to be released. It is okay to say goodbye little by little, but for total healing, we eventually must completely let go.
Begin by substituting certain ingredients in your favorite recipes with the intention of complete transformation. Just the thought of replacing your mom's Italian style 'Spaghetti Bolognese' with vegan tofu-nese at first seems disgusting but after you try it (prepare it yourself the first time) you will enjoy every bite.
Once again, you may want to research other sources for ideas and tips for this transition.

Suggestions and tips to ease discomfort during transitioning...
        Allow and accept what is. Changing our way of life, we will at first experience challenges and uncomfortable situations. Once we decide to accept whatever is happening as a part of our necessary experience on this journey, a light begins to shine within and we feel lighter and happier.
Maintain your daily practice of yoga, meditation, or any other discipline to improve your awareness and focus.
Be kind and compassionate with yourself and remember that a lifetime of abusing our body, minds, and spirits cannot heal overnight.
Enjoy the process and bear in mind that the rewards you will reap are beyond measure.

'Those who act with bravery and courage will overcome diseases, while those who act out of fear will fall ill.'
The Yellow Emperor's Classic of Internal Medicine

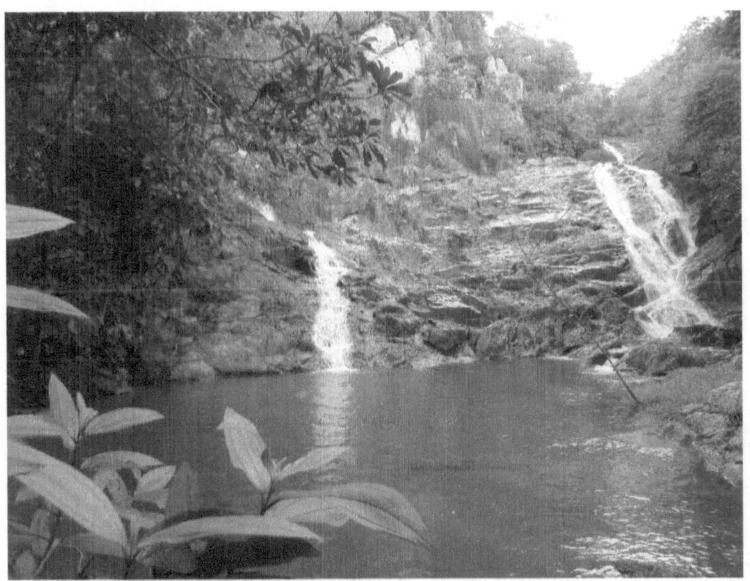

CHAPTER 5   ENCOURAGEMENT

'My parents did not always agree with my life choices but that did not stop them from their understanding and support in whatever it was I chose as my path. They never stopped loving me no matter what my life's direction. For this I am most grateful and have found real happiness.' Anonymous

Encouragement - from the French… Genuine heartfelt support of another's efforts of achieving a difficult task. Any journey in this human life whether it is an

adventurous trek to distant lands or a spiritual quest of the inner world is made less challenging through the genuine support and encouragement from family and friends who wish to see you succeed. When one is blessed to have this kind of support the journey is less arduous.

Ways to ease possible resistance or aversion to your new lifestyle from family and friends include;

CHAPTER 6   RE-TREAT YOURSELF

Re-Treat Yourself

Attending a workshop, seminar, or special retreat for the purpose of enriching your life is a wonderful way to grow in conscious awareness. Besides the added knowledge and techniques you will gain, socializing with like-minded people is tremendously beneficial and inspiring. Exchanging thoughts and ideas… Networking and making new friends is invaluable for our progress on the path.

However, if you are even the least bit disciplined, you can do it yourself right where you are. You can design your own personal retreat in your own home. To be effective and powerful, a home based 'Retreat' needs to be just that... A retreat from the daily norm with no distractions including interruptions from family, phone calls, or door bells. The practice must be scheduled and occur as close as possible to the same time every day. A special space is necessary and should be free of distraction and noise. Your daily morning practice can be anywhere you choose. Have it be a sacred space and someplace where you feel nourished. Early morning is an optimal time for a spiritual practice, whether it is Meditation, Yoga, Chanting, or any other type of life-enriching activity. Family support and encouragement makes your home retreat that much more effective and rewarding. Don't forget to take advantage of all the videos available on the internet. Many of them are free and some can be downloaded for a reasonable price.

CHAPTER 7   WATER...WATER...

 'When the well is dry, we will know the worth of water.'
Benjamin Franklin

The importance of clean, pure water cannot be

overstated. This is the reason for a whole chapter

dedicated to this essential food.

Emphasis is made here on this precious natural

resource because of it's prominent role in the natural

healing process. Water is the world's first and foremost

medicine. This life sustaining liquid makes up over two-

thirds of our body's mass and maintaing this level

especially while we are in transition to a healing diet is absolutely essential. Old stored toxins and residues in the body require an abundance of water to be effectively flushed out of our system during this restorative process. Pure, clean drinking water is a life sustaining nutrient for all life on planet Earth. The quality of our drinking water is therefore of the utmost importance. In a perfect world, all beings would have access to pure, fresh, and clean drinking water. However, as it is, millions upon millions of the worlds inhabitants have little or no access to pure, potable water. And... to make a sad situation worse, privatization of community water reservoirs by multinational corporations is increasing at an astonishing rate. The quality of the water is diminishing as well as the service and in many communities, the costs to the poor consumer is rising at an alarming rate. So much so that many can no longer afford to buy water and are forced to use water from polluted rivers and other waterways. The disease and related deaths from this practice are going unreported and virtually nothing is being done to reverse this insidious practice by corporations... all for the sake of profit.

'Thousands have lived without love...not one without water.' W H Auden

So... for those of us fortunate enough to still have the luxury of turning on the faucet and drawing potable water, we can be truly grateful and remind ourselves to never take this for granted. That being said, even in well to do communities, the water coming out of the spigot is not safe for drinking. Chlorine, fluoride and who knows what other toxic chemicals are widely present in community water reservoirs. Chlorine has been for years labeled as toxic to all living beings, but yet there it is... in our drinking water. Chlorine combines with other organic substance in water and forms chloroform which is a poisonous chemical, known to cause cancer. Fluoride has been added to the municipal water supplies since after the second world war supposedly to help prevent tooth decay. Originally, tooth decay prevention tests were performed with calcium fluoride, however the chemical compound present in municipal water supplies prevalent in the US is sodium fluoride and fluorisilicic acid, by products of the farming and chemical fertilizer industry and are highly contaminated with lead and arsenic. Hard to believe, but until the practice of adding this poisonous chemical to the public water supply was instituted by the US government, the primary use for fluoride was as a rat poison? In many European countries, including Germany, Holland, Denmark, Sweden, Norway, Belgium, and France, fluoride is illegal in their metropolitan water supplies.

'In an age when man has forgotten his origins and is blind even to his most essential needs for survival, clean water has become the victim of his indifference.'
Rachel Carson

What are our alternatives?

Distilled water is water that has been boiled into steam and condensed back into liquid in a separate container. Impurities in the original water that do not boil below or at the boiling point of water remain in the original container. Thus, distilled water is one type of purified water.

Activated charcoal filters are a popular method of removing most wastes and toxins that are not water soluble from drinking water.

Reverse osmosis purifiers do pretty much the same thing but at a greater cost to the consumer.

Bottled water is even a more expensive alternative to filtered water but some high quality bottled spring waters are available from France, Iceland, Germany and Italy. These waters are from natural sources and maintain their purity and mineral content.

Private and rural wells are not as safe these days especially if they are near agricultural areas which are farming organically. Have your water tested regularly to insure it is free of contaminates.

Mountain streams are also sketchy sources of clean water in these times. If you are using water from a mountain stream it should also be tested.
Springs and underground aquifers were at one time a crystal clear and pure source of drinking water and were common place. These natural sources of drinking water are diminishing rapidly either because they have dried up from extreme weather changes or more commonly

have been contaminated by chemical pollutants or have been sold to 'For profit' corporations.

A reliable and tested source of pure, mountain spring water is valuable beyond measure. We are fortunate in that where we are living in Europe only a short drive away is a precious, clean source of spring water. The spring is tested quarterly for any bacteria or contaminants and has been for many years. The water source is in a protected natural area and for the time being, is free for those who wish to use it. We are intent on maintaining these conditions as long as possible. I never thought I would have such gratitude for water, but I do and I will never take it for granted.

Be thankful for any clean, pure source of water available to you. Think of the hundreds of millions of Earth's inhabitants of who have little or no source of potable water and are yet grateful to just be alive.

CHAPTER 8   COMMUNE WITH NATURE

'A kiss of the sun for pardon… A song of the birds for mirth… One is nearer God's heart in a garden than anywhere else on Earth.'
Dorothy Frances Gurney

The Healing Power of Nature

Through regularly connecting with the natural world we gain a stronger sense of our own magnificence. Wandering on a forest path, or strolling along an ocean beach… Sitting in a quiet garden admiring the flowers or hiking a mountain trail… all contribute to nourishing our spirit. Being in nature, we have the opportunity to reconnect to our true essence if we are quiet and feel with our hearts and not our minds. A whole new world opens up before us when we connect energetically with not just the natural world but with all of life.

When we look with the innocent eyes of a child, we see what is really there and not what we conceive as being there from past experiences and encounters. We do not automatically identify and label this tree, that flower, or those birds or other creatures. Have you ever watched a baby just staring unblinkingly as if in complete awe at what is seen? There is no mind nor thinking or comparing happening... only pure seeing for the first time. If we could cultivate this characteristic as adult humans then a whole new world would open up for us. We would regain that awe for life we had as a child.

My wife and I are fortunate to live within walking and biking distance to a vast wilderness preserve thick with mature trees and lush vegetation. Within minutes of entering, any existing stress or tension begins to melt away. Often we sit and meditate and afterwards feel a sense of relaxation and regeneration. The healing and nourishing benefits from a leisurely stroll in a natural environment such as a forest, lake, ocean, or other natural environments are, needless to say, a powerful

antidote to the stress of normal, everyday life. If you do not have the luxury of living close to a wilderness area or ocean beach and are living in a city perhaps you can visit the municipal park or pedestrian mall which normally provide some quiet, natural areas.
Natural environments are a truly nourishing place to revitalize and calm our busy minds and stressed out bodies.

'Every morning was a cheerful invitation to make my life of equal simplicity, and I may say innocence with Nature herself.' Henry David Thoreau

CHAPTER 9   HEALTH ASSURANCE

'Security is mostly a superstition. It does not exist in nature, nor do the children of men as a whole experience it. Avoiding danger is no safer in the long run than outright exposure. Life is either a daring adventure or nothing. To keep our faces turned towards change and behave like free spirits in the presence of fate is strength undefeatable. Helen Keller

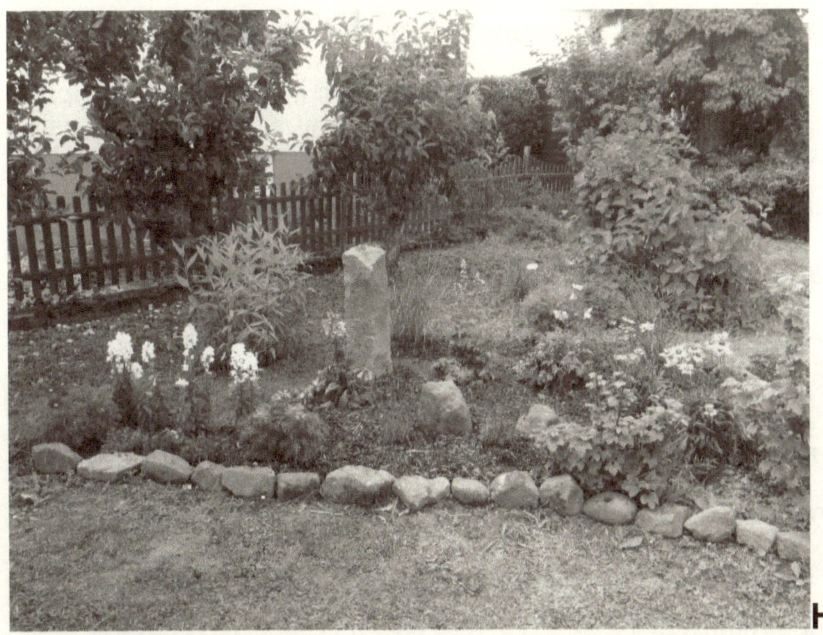

ealth Assurance

Nothing in this life is certain and everything is in a constant state of flux. Most of the time, it may appear as though there is security in our lives and we are in control, but the truth is, as Helen Keller so succinctly said, 'Security is mostly a superstition'. Look around and try to find 'Security' in the natural world. It simply does not exist. We can avoid disaster and improve our chances of living a healthy life simply by asking ourselves in each moment, 'Is what I am about to do nourishing me or is it harming me'. Pausing with a few deep breaths and listening with the heart is a sure fire solution to making the right choices in every situation. Guaranteed!

Vibrant, great health and vitality are an invaluable benefit from taking your personal well being into your own hands through wholesome living. Besides this and numerous other advantages there is the possibility of saving thousands of dollars a year on health insurance premiums. This is not a recommendation to cancel your Health Insurance Policy but to perhaps consider other possibilities.

Due in part to the increase in severe and chronic illnesses in the US, the costs of insurances premiums continue to soar and not just for those at risk of serious illness, but for those of us who are diligently taking good care of our own personal health. Presently across America, it is estimated that more than 46 million people are without health insurance. Another 40 million have inadequate health coverage. This means that nearly one-third of all Americans face each day living in fear of the possibility of falling ill or needing a doctor in an emergency and having not the resources to do anything about it. Often, an otherwise treatable symptom or sickness develops into a tragedy when families avoid seeing a doctor because they cannot afford it. And when they absolutely are forced to visit the emergency room or doctor's office, (if the doctor will see the patient at all) some basic necessity or other will have to be sacrificed to pay the exorbitant medical fees. This is quite common, especially in the United States, but now it is increasing in other parts of the world. Consider the fact that most of the Earth's inhabitants live their entire lives with no type of Health care whatsoever.

Change is Coming

In surprising numbers, people across America, having finally had enough of costly doctor's bills, ridiculously expensive medications, corporate greed, and the lack of incentives being offered by health insurers to stay healthy, are taking matters into their own hands. The rise in the number of individuals, entire families, and in some cases whole communities, instituting healthier lifestyles is considerable and quite inspiring to see. This trend can only grow as awareness of Healthy Living continues its spread. At the forefront of this movement are young people realizing that the government, corporations, the medical profession, and the pharmaceutical industry care for no one but themselves and their profits. They are educating themselves about good nutrition, proper daily exercise, and mental and spiritual health.

A good sign of the changing times are the small but growing numbers of newer health insurance start-ups offering lower premiums for health conscious individuals and families. Health IQ in San Diego California is offering special life insurance rates for Vegans... and the trend of consideration for those of us making every effort to life a truly healthy life continues. Israeli health insurance company, Clal Insurance, is offering discounted health insurance to Vegans who qualify through presenting a 'declaration of health'. For most people, the mere thought of living with no Health care is a very scary scenario and rightly so. Financial ruin could happen in an instant through some catastrophic illness or accident. All the more reason to take the responsibility of our personal 'Health care' back and increase our chances of never needing to rely on someone or some entity outside of ourselves to heal us. What a tremendous sense of self-empowerment we acquire when we begin to experience a strengthened immune system, increased energy and vitality, and self confidence through having taken back control of our personal health and well being.

By following simple and practical guidelines and developing and sharpening our intuitive abilities, we increase our wisdom and knowledge of self-healing. We begin to live our lives authentically and honestly and… the added benefit of inspiring those around us through being a good example and thus creating a community of like-minded people.

This is but a tiny glimpse of what the future holds for us on the planet Earth. Contrary to what the Corporations,

Governments, Politicians, and Religions would have us believe, a new and powerful consciousness is arising now. One that will be independent from the whims of all of those who would have us conform to their greedy, selfish agendas. The age of truth is, at last, upon us and is growing stronger - person by person… day by day and is here to stay for a long, long time.

Modern western medicine must be recognized for its remarkable skill in treating emergency situations without which, many of us would have had a very short life.

CHAPTER 10 MANIFESTING A RICH LIFE

'The greatest and most valuable things in this life are given to us freely. Vibrant, good health, happiness, and freedom.' Anonymous

Manifesting A Rich Life

If any among us wishes to learn the true meaning of the word 'Abundance' then a visit to India or other 'Third world' country would be a valuable opportunity to learn this and of course many other important life lessons. After my time in India, I have become much more grateful for the simple things and conveniences of my everyday life. I no longer equate the word 'Abundance' with prosperity or material wealth. True abundance, I have discovered, has absolutely nothing to do with material wealth or prosperity. For most of the people living on this Earth, an abundant life means having enough, period...

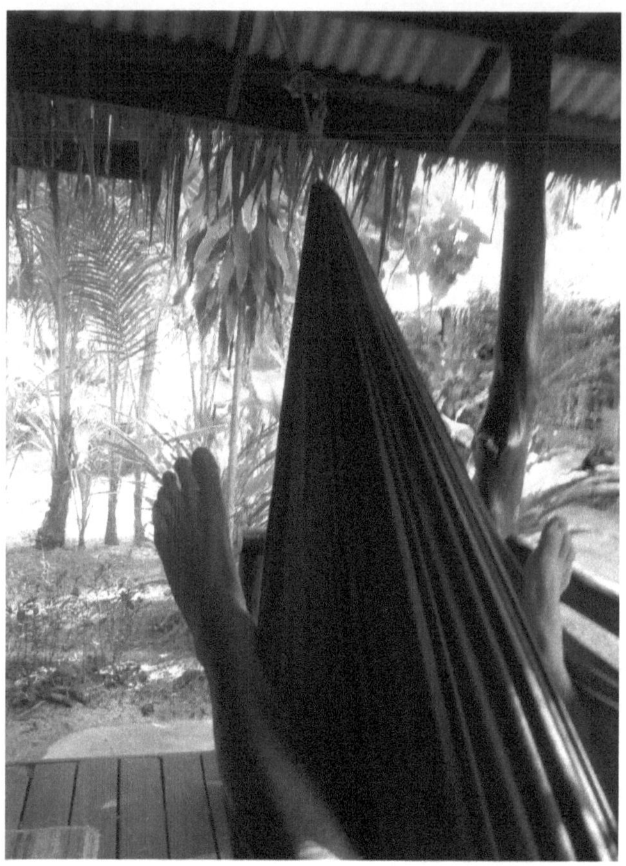

Vibrant, good health for oneself and family… Fresh air
to breathe… Clean water to drink and to bathe in...
Food enough for the whole family to be nourished.
A warm, dry place to lay one's head at night.
These are the simple, basic necessities for which many
of us take for granted while we strive for the
'unnecessary' even excessive 'worldly goods' which
ultimately take us away from true abundance and
gratefulness. Visiting a third world country like India

could surely help but is not necessary. We can begin to

value the everyday, basic things for which we take for

granted through simply being grateful. By pausing

before a meal and consider the farmer who worked to

grow the food. For the sun and the rain and the soil. For

those who helped to make it available to us. And for

those who lovingly prepared it. For all of the things in

our lives which we would normally take for granted, if

we just take a moment to consider what life would be

without these precious gifts, and offer a simple prayer of

thanks, then our lives will

become truly abundant.

'Our goal on this Earth is to mature to the point where
we no longer need the experiences of the material world
for development.'

Being absolutely clear about what it is you want is the

first step. As soon you make a conscious decision to

change your life for the better, you attract to you the

creative powers of the Universe which will support you

in manifesting your dream. Contrary to what we've been

led to believe regarding creating abundance… Hard work, sweat, and sacrifice is absolutely not necessary to achieve this goal. Pure and simple… Intention, strong will, and a clear vision are the only ingredients you need to achieve your dreams. And there are many methods to do this without sacrificing your health and well being. Prayer, meditation, visualisations, chanting, creating a vision board, and so on.

Once you are clear what it is you wish to manifest in your life then give it out to the Universe, God, or whatever higher power you believe in and trust that your dreams will be realized. However, it is absolutely essential that you be as specific as possible otherwise you may not like the form in which your dreams become manifest.

Important points to remember:

Voice your wishes and dreams aloud. They become instantly transformed from a simple idea (spirit world) into the beginnings of a reality (physical world). Further physicalization can be writing down paper your specific dreams or wishes.

Do something every day towards your goal. Have a vision board or reminder posted in several places around your home where you will see it daily.

Trust in the process. Realize that it may take time. Have patience.

Accept and acknowledge whatever it is you receive even if it is different than what you imagined. It is all part of the process.

Maintain a healthy, pure lifestyle. Keep you energy and vibration high and continue to raise your frequency so that it continues to vibrate at a higher and higher level. Completely let go of any resistance for the changes occurring in your life. Whatever is happening is all part of the process of realizing your goal.

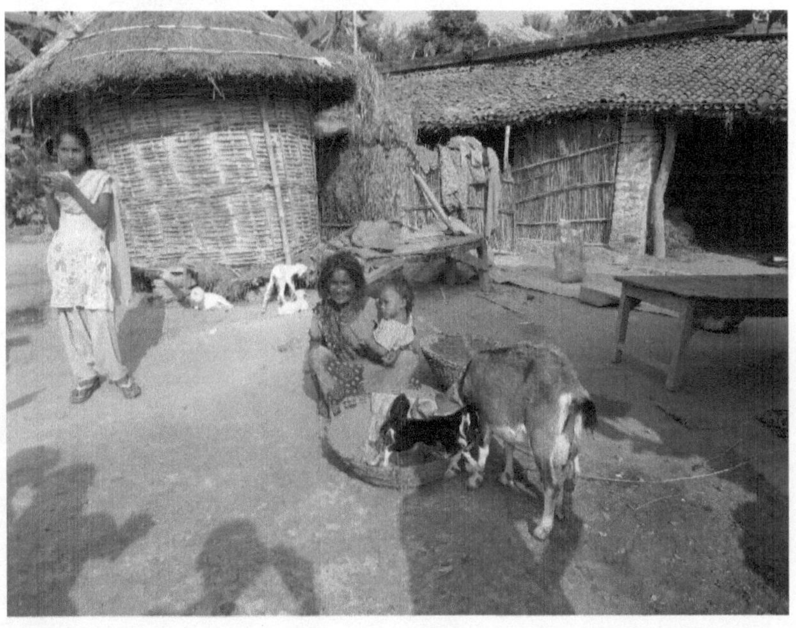

'All progress, all fulfillment of desire depends on the control and concentration of your attention.'   Neville Goddard

Manifesto: The Mad Farmer Liberation Front
by Wendell Berry

Love the quick profit, the annual raise,
vacation with pay. Want more
of everything ready-made. Be afraid
to know your neighbors and to die.
And you will have a window in your head.
Not even your future will be a mystery
any more. Your mind will be punched in a card
and shut away in a little drawer.
When they want you to buy something
they will call you. When they want you
to die for profit they will let you know.
So, friends, every day do something
that won't compute. Love the Lord.
Love the world. Work for nothing.
Take all that you have and be poor.
Love someone who does not deserve it.
Denounce the government and embrace
the flag. Hope to live in that free
republic for which it stands.
Give your approval to all you cannot
understand. Praise ignorance, for what man
has not encountered he has not destroyed.
Ask the questions that have no answers.
Invest in the millennium. Plant sequoias.
Say that your main crop is the forest
that you did not plant,

that you will not live to harvest.
Say that the leaves are harvested
when they have rotted into the mold.
Call that profit. Prophesy such returns.
Put your faith in the two inches of humus
that will build under the trees
every thousand years.
Listen to carrion — put your ear
close, and hear the faint chattering
of the songs that are to come.
Expect the end of the world. Laugh.
Laughter is immeasurable. Be joyful
though you have considered all the facts.
So long as women do not go cheap
for power, please women more than men.
Ask yourself: Will this satisfy
a woman satisfied to bear a child?
Will this disturb the sleep
of a woman near to giving birth?
Go with your love to the fields.
Lie easy in the shade. Rest your head
in her lap. Swear allegiance
to what is nighest your thoughts.
As soon as the generals and the politicos
can predict the motions of your mind,
lose it. Leave it as a sign
to mark the false trail, the way
you didn't go. Be like the fox
who makes more tracks than necessary,
some in the wrong direction.
Practice resurrection.

'No greeter sin than desire. No greater curse than discontent. No greater misfortune than wanting something for oneself. Therefore, she who knows that enough is enough will always have enough.' Lao Tsu

CHAPTER 11   PASS IT ON

'A single moment can change the day, a single day can change an entire life, a single life can change the entire world'. Buddha

Pass It On

Being an inspiration to others is not as difficult as we would think. For several years now, we've been experimenting with gently sharing our love, compassion, and understanding with others just by being present and aware. Through direct, personal experience, we have witnessed immediate, spontaneous changes in peoples' demeanors when we offer, genuinely and from the heart, a smile, a kind word or a simple gesture of caring. No matter where we are or with whom we interact, being present and smiling to everyone we meet kindles a light in even the most disconsolate individuals. Almost all will respond and smile back because you have touched their heart of hearts and… no matter how fortified or closed, the heart almost always opens up and receives the authentic love and kindness it is being offered.

The feeling which is awakened in those we have touched with our love and kindness spreads from one person to the other and we never really know how many lives we have touched in a positive way.

Sharing kindness, compassion, and understanding is an effective method of demonstrating to others a way of being that is not always focused on what is 'Not right' with the world. Instead, a spark of light is ignited within them and they have a glimpse of the 'Goodness' that is all around them all of the time.

Furthermore… Sharing knowledge and wisdom with others, when it comes from our hearts and when we expect nothing in return is a truly powerful gift. It is the most genuine and valuable action we can make towards inspiring others to begin to walk the path towards 'Self-realization.

It has been said that we are merely vehicles through which the creative powers of God, the Universe, the Life Force, or whatever one chooses to name 'It' are 'transmitted'. Many of the beloved and inspiring individuals from the past and of the present times have shared their wisdom and knowledge with no thought of reward or remuneration of any kind. They understand intuitively that the wisdom and knowledge imparted to them was not theirs, that they did not own this wisdom nor did they have exclusive rights to it, instead, it was gifted to them for the purpose of benefitting from it and then passing it on to anyone who wished to know and understand the true value of these ancient wisdom teachings.

When we are in a state of high consciousness… in a places of calm and present moment awareness, we are able to 'Tune in' to these Ancient wisdom teachings'. This energy is around us all of the time and is always available to any being who is truly seeking to 'Wake up' to Life.

Those who have come before us and who have also walked this very same path towards liberation endured much more challenges and pitfalls to get where we are with much less effort. To be grateful for their efforts and their progress almost entirely on their own and of their own volition is an honourable way to respect what we have been given freely. Recognizing our predecessors for their endeavours and challenges is the highest form of the art of

This does not mean we worship anyone or hold them is such high esteem that we forget who, at our very essence, we truly are… a divine being, inextricably interconnected to the creative power of the universe.

'Be the change you want to see in the world'.

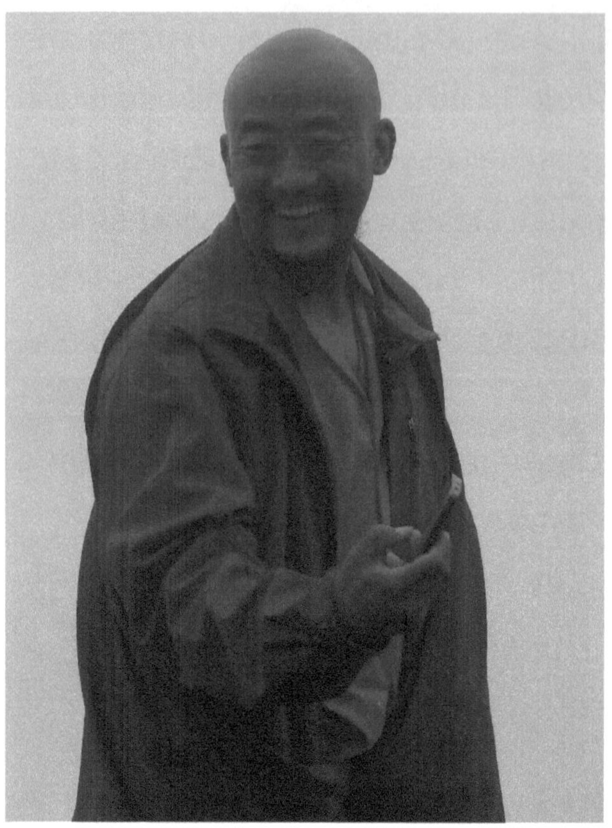

CHAPTER 12   GRATITUDE

Tis a gift to be simple,
'Tis a gift to be free,
'Tis a gift to come down where we ought to be,
And when we find ourselves in the place just right,
It will be in the valley of love and delight.
When true simplicity is gained,
to bow and to bend, we will not be ashamed
To turn, turn, will be our delight,
'Til by turning, turning, we come round right. Shaker
song

Gratitude

Thankfulness is a subtle but powerful energy which appears to flow forth from the human heart. It is pure and alive and can affect our life in ways which cannot be fathomed or measured. Gratitude can occur naturally, It can arise from the awareness of all of the abundance in our lives… no matter how grand or how simple. Sometimes being grateful comes from great suffering or a life threatening experience. What a blessing it is when pure gratefulness flows forth from your heart with only the realization that you are alive. Every day is a brand new day… A precious gift… and when we feel this marvelous, warm glow of gratitude, we begin to notice all around us the wondrous miracle of life. We open our eyes as for the first time and delight in the quiet beauty of the natural world… we hear with our ears, the joyous song of the birds… the pure, innocence of laughing children… with our sense of smell, the fresh sweet fragrance of the forest soil… all this and more fills us with a feeling of joyous gratitude for this human experience.

We have so much to be grateful for. At this time on planet Earth, so much suffering, chaos and confusion make it difficult for us to focus on what is right and good and wonderful. If we can turn away from the negative and dwell on the positive, we change not only our own energy, but the energy of those around us. To be grateful for our life, no matter how simple, is a powerful force which can have a far reaching effect. Begin each morning with thankfulness for this new day because although we often take it for granted, it is not just another day in your life. It is a brand new day. It is a precious gift given to us to enjoy… to be happy and to share this happiness with many others. When we do this and it comes from a genuine place in our hearts then we change in miraculous ways and the world suddenly becomes a beautiful place. Happiness really is the result of being truly grateful and not the other way around.

Authentic, joyful gratitude is an invisible force which touches everyone and everything around you. You emanate peace and calm and this energy is contagious affecting all beings.

Cultivate genuine gratitude, notice the things in your life for which you take for granted… and for which most of the world will never experience… for this is one of the most powerful ways to effect positive change in our world.

'I am grateful for what I am and have. My thanksgiving is perpetual.'

Henry David Thoreau

Charles Kuhn (Stone) and Monika Schneider (Stone) are teaching, writing, and farming in the foothills of the Blue Ridge mountains of Virginia.
Based on the premise that we can leave this Earth better than we found it, Monika & Charles are making it their life's work to first rejuvenate and revitalize the living soil from which we all derive our sustenance. They are sharing the abundant harvests from their gardens with family, friends, and the community. Through living by example, a more loving, wholesome, and nourishing life, they feel certain many others will want the same.
Being close to Nature and through practicing the Arts of Simple Living and Self Sufficiency, we are bound to become whole, happy human beings.

May the long time Sun shine upon you.
May all the Love in the Universe surround you.

Contact;
Charles@EarthWise.Live
Monika@EarthWise.Live
or visit our website:
www.EarthWise.Live